TRACE ELEMENTS

TRACE ELEMENTS

Miracle Micro Nutrients

Dr Andrew Stanway

THORSONS PUBLISHING GROUP
Wellingborough, Northamptonshire
———— · ————
Rochester, Vermont

First published by Van Dyke Books Ltd. 1983
This revised edition 1987

British Library Cataloguing in Publication Data

Stanway, Andrew
Trace elements: miracle micro nutrients
in nutrients. —— 2nd ed.
1. Trace elements in nutrition
I. Title
613.2'8   TX553.T7

ISBN 0-7225-1157-4

Printed in Great Britain by Richard Clay Ltd, Bungay, Suffolk

1 3 5 7 9 10 8 6 4 2

CONTENTS

CHAPTER ONE

INTRODUCTION

HISTORY

Over the last 25 years or so, following almost a century of scientific pre-occupation with the study of vitamins, an interest has grown up in the minerals that are important in the body's healthy functioning. This has led to a relatively new scientific discipline, bio-inorganic chemistry, that deals with the non-living building blocks of living things. At first one could be forgiven for thinking that because the substances being studied are 'chemicals' as opposed to living body structures (such as cells), they'd be easy to study. Alas, this is far from the truth—mainly because these seemingly simple substances, once incorporated into the body of an animal or human, become part of an extremely intricate system or, more accurately, a collection of inter-linked systems, the complexity of which still almost entirely baffles us.

The Greeks realized that rusty iron left in water made the water a useful cure for anaemia, and iodine has been known to cure goitre for hundreds of years, but until recently the non-living (inorganic) substances of the body had been little studied and even less understood.

As with so many areas of modern medicine, animal nutritionists and veterinarians have led the way. The father of our modern understanding of this area was the Australian animal nutritionist Dr E. J. Underwood FRS, who first described a deficiency of the essential mineral cobalt in the 1930s. Until he died in 1980 he was a pioneer in both veterinary and human mineral nutrition. The financial pressures to get things right in animal husbandry (with the enormous sums of money involved in this sort of farming) are so great that research is soon done to find the causes of diseases and disorders in animals. The human population has no parallel watchdog and many of us undoubtedly suffer (as we shall see in the book) from nutritional imbalances which would have been understood and treated long ago had we been farm animals!

But today things are changing rapidly and with lessons learned from animal husbandry an exciting new chapter is opening up in modern nutrition. However, although there has been a lot of research in humans over the last quarter of a century, little of it has found its way into clinical medicine and many, if not most, doctors are very wary of the subject.

This book will, I hope, shed some light on this important if, as yet, ill-understood area of nutrition, and so help us to live more healthy lives.

WHAT ARE TRACE ELEMENTS?

A chemical 'element' is, technically speaking, a non-living (inorganic) substance that consists of atoms with the same number of protons in its nucleus. There are 105 known elements (nature's basic building blocks) in the universe, of which 93 are naturally-occurring and the others man-made. All living, and non-living, things are made up of these 93 chemical substances arranged in an infinite variety of ways.

At the present time 27 elements are known to be essential for life. Besides the 11 major elements, carbon (C), hydrogen (H), oxygen (O), nitrogen (N), sulphur (S), calcium (Ca), phosphorus (P), potassium (K), sodium (Na), chlorine (Cl) and magnesium (Mg), there are 16 others that are accepted as essential for mammals in general and Man in particular. These are iron (Fe), zinc (Zn), copper (Cu), manganese (Mn), nickel (Ni), cobalt (Co), molybdenum (Mo), selenium (Se), chromium (Cr), iodine (I), fluorine (F), tin (Sn), silicon (Si), vanadium (V), and perhaps surprisingly in view of our preoccupation with their toxicity, arsenic (As) and lead (Pb). Of these 16 trace elements, 10 are considered to be the most important and essential clinically. These are copper, iron, zinc, cobalt, iodine, molybdenum, manganese, selenium, chromium and fluorine.

The amounts of the first 11 of the 27 elements in the body are large and have been measurable for decades. However, the amounts of the other 16 are (apart from iron) very tiny indeed. Because they are present only in the tiniest traces (measured in parts per million or parts per billion) they have come to be called 'trace' elements. Although the term 'trace element' gives an impression of inaccuracy—rather like a 'pinch' of salt—this is far from the case in reality. The study and measurement of these trace elements is now a subject of considerable interest to the medical and veterinary professions and there are tens of thousands of learned papers on the subject in the scientific literature around the world.

Of course, it isn't simply enough to say that because there is a trace of an element in the body that it is essential for life—after all it could be a contaminant or a toxin. As a result, a lot of trace element research has put great stress on defining the 'essential' nature of these substances. After all, unless they can be proven to be essential for life their importance recedes in value. If we had sufficiently accurate measuring methods we could probably find all 93 naturally-occurring elements in the body, but to claim that they were necessary for health might be quite wrong.

There are several ways of defining 'essentiality' but we'll just look at the three main ones here. First, one could define an element as essential if its deficiency resulted in an impairment of function of the person or animal involved—the degree of dysfunction being related to the degree of deficiency. Clearly evidence for such work must come from animals because it would be totally unethical to feed humans diets grossly deficient in certain elements to see what signs and symptoms were produced. Such work *has* been done in animals and forms the basis of our understanding of the trace element deficiency diseases.

A second way of defining essentiality is to ask oneself what the substance is essential for. Essential for growth? Essential for pregnancy and lactation? Essential for reproduction? This becomes important because some elements are essential during early life (before maturity) but later appear to play only a minor role, whilst for other elements the reverse is true.

But a more stringent definition of essentiality insists on several criteria being fulfilled. First, the element must be present in healthy tissues of all organisms; second, its concentrations in these tissues should be relatively constant; and third, its withdrawal should always produce similar structural and physiological abnormalities which are prevented or reversed by the addition of the element. Obviously for an element to be essential, its removal must produce an ill-effect which can be remedied by returning it.

This discussion on essentiality is crucial because there have already been so many red herrings in medicine (and particularly in nutrition) that it would be inexcusable to encourage people to worry about, for example, their zinc status, if it could be proved that zinc wasn't necessary for the body but was simply a contaminant from the environment.

WHERE DO THEY COME FROM?

To understand the dietary sources of trace elements we need first to look briefly at the dietary history of Man.

Man as we know him has evolved slowly from his primate ancestors who lived on the fringes of tropical forests about 3 million years ago. Such early hominids were undoubtedly mainly vegetarians but became increasingly omnivorous. This dietary change came about because of climatic alterations that reduced the extent of the rain forest and produced enormous areas of savannah and grasslands that supported rich herds of grazing animals. With the discovery and invention of implements, fires and cooking, Man was beginning to be able to hunt, cook and store food and so enjoyed a varied and balanced omnivorous diet. With the coming of agriculture about 15,000 years ago cereals derived from the wild grasses that dominated the inhabited world became the main source of food for Man and his animals. This could be seen as a return to being dependent on plant food sources.

Archaeologists in the U.S. and Europe have looked at the history of diet and their researches have shed much light on the importance of trace elements. Studies of the Indian inhabitation sites in the Kentucky blue grass area, for example, have shown how trace elements have shaped Man's development over the centuries. There, the soil content was very suitable for grazing animals and the people followed their animals. But with the introduction of agriculture a sedentary population was established. Soon the people started to suffer from dental and bony abnormalities (as judged by human remains). Here, and in other archaeological sites, bones and teeth have provided excellent evidence of the trace element status of peoples who lived thousands of years ago. Such remains are especially useful for studying zinc, copper and magnesium. The zinc content of bone can tell us with some accuracy what proportion of meat to vegetables a population consumed, and the proportion of magnesium to zinc can give some guide as to the trends in nutrition over several generations.

The trace elements occur in human blood in amounts which can be correlated very closely with the proportions found in the earth's crust—indeed all trace elements come originally from the soil. Whether we end up inhaling them in some form of dust (which is especially plentiful in urban areas), drinking them in water, or eating them in food will depend very much on where we live and what we eat. Suffice it to say that for most people food is the most important source of trace elements. Water, however, is not a negligible source, as was once thought and we shall look at this on page 17. The other main sources are from plant and animal foods and these are considered in detail on pages 19-25.

WHAT DO TRACE ELEMENTS DO?

During the last 25 years enormous progress has been made in understanding how the trace elements work within the body's tissues and how they are transported around the body. This has been made possible by using radioactively labelled elements which are injected or taken orally. These follow the path of the naturally-occurring trace elements in the body but can be detected readily because of their radioactive 'tag'. The discovery of many metal-containing proteins with enzymatic activity has also shed a lot of light on trace element metabolism, mainly because most of these proteins need trace elements in their production. But perhaps the greatest steps forward have come as a result of very precise and sensitive measuring techniques that make the measurement of substances present in parts per million or billion not only possible but affordable and relatively straightforward.

Just as vitamins are unique chemical entities which are 'keys' to unique biological 'locks' in any given situation, so the same is true of the trace elements. As far as we know, no trace element can be replaced by another, although some can displace others and so render them useless.

Many trace elements are now known to work because of their crucial role in the structure of enzymes—the body's activator systems that make every process of life function normally. They are also needed for the transport of essential nutrients around the body, for tissue formation and for bone formation. Several individual trace elements are now known to be crucial for the formation of RNA and DNA—the substances at the heart of life itself within any cell. In contrast to this almost universal necessity there are other none the less essential trace elements such as iodine and cobalt whose significance seems to be to one body system only (the thyroid and vitamin B_{12} metabolism respectively). Most trace elements fall somewhere between these two extremes.

The way a trace element works varies with its level in the body, as we have seen already. The biological range of dose produces health; the pharmacological dose puts right any deficiency there may be; and at higher levels the toxic dose causes signs of trouble and even death. For most trace elements the range of safety is extremely wide, far more so than for other nutrients in the body. This is probably because the body has, for many elements, the capacity to regulate absorption and excretion according to demand and in some instances has the additional ability to store any excess in the form of harmless deposits in certain tissues.

For some trace elements, however, the differences between the minimal essential concentration in the diet or in the environment, and the maximum that the body can tolerate is very narrow. Selenium and fluorine are good examples. Such elements are often thought of as mainly toxic when in fact within a very limited range of intake they are essential.

The body's needs for trace elements, and to some extent the way it handles them, depend greatly on its state at the time. So stress caused by infection, injury, an operation, pregnancy, a hormone imbalance or the excessive intake of a particular food may show up a relative deficiency of a trace element that would otherwise be masked. It is now known that certain cell and body systems put particular demands on the total pool of trace elements in the body at different times of life and in different pathological conditions. So a seemingly well woman in apparent balance for say zinc, could become zinc-deficient during pregnancy or during prolonged breast-feeding.

Delicate processes keep a balance between the body's stores of trace elements, the blood (which transports them) and the tissues where they are needed. Sophisticated control systems balance all these out in a healthy person so that when we eat a meal very rich in a particular element it will either not be absorbed at all (if the body has plenty of it) or it will be absorbed and taken to storage tissues (often in the liver) until the body needs more of it.

Lastly, while on the subject of how trace elements work, we should look at interactions arising between individual elements because these are now recognized as very important, and because trace elements seem to be more susceptible to dietary and environmental influences than most of the body's substances generally. If one is zinc-deficient, then this is made worse if the intake of calcium or copper is high. In contrast, tolerance of excessive lead or cadmium is markedly reduced if tissue reserves of calcium, phosphorus, zinc or iron are low. Sometimes trace elements interact with food to produce complex chemical compounds which aren't absorbed; sometimes one element competes with another for the transport mechanism across the intestinal wall into the bloodstream; and there are doubtless other mechanisms that are as yet undiscovered. The importance of such processes affecting the availability of the trace elements is wisely appreciated in crop husbandry and farm animal nutrition. So clearly, trace element nutrition is subtle and can't be looked at in quite the same way as our needs for other essential 'nutrients'. At one end of the scale we can last only a few minutes without oxygen. At the other are the trace elements in which deficiencies take some time to become apparent and simply giving more of the one that appears to be in short supply may not be the answer.

THE CLASSIFICATION OF TRACE ELEMENTS

Once we have agreed that 10 elements are essential, how can we group them to help us understand them better? Frankly, it's very difficult but an arbitrary classification could run as follows:

1. Trace elements with reported beneficial effects in Man: chromium, cobalt, copper, iodine, molybdenum, selenium, and zinc.

2. Trace elements with beneficial effects so far established only in lower species of animals: manganese.

3. Trace elements whose biological effects are more usually related to excessive intake: molybdenum.

The problem with any such classification is that it gives the impression that there are clear dividing lines between the groups. This is not necessarily so. For example, whilst it might be assumed that it would be a simple matter to decide whether a trace element is toxic (poisonous) or not in the body, the truth is very different. All trace elements are toxic if taken in large enough amounts and tiny traces of some elements previously thought to be poisonous (such as arsenic) are now thought to be essential for life. It is also a characteristic of trace elements that their toxicity varies profoundly according to the chemical form of the element. Also, the safe dietary level of any one trace element is intimately linked to the concentration of the others and also affects their absorption and retention in the body. So, for example, the relative intake of zinc, iron and copper can determine whether signs of copper deficiency or toxicity occur. Similarly, arsenic has been found to be the best dietary factor to reduce selenium toxicity in animals, and so on.

Each trace element then has several levels at which it works in the body as we can see from Figure 1. If there is none present, death or disease will ensue, as they will if there is a massive overdose. At the lower end of the scale signs of deficiency will occur but as the levels rise these may be hidden or not clinically apparent. In the centre section of the graph the person is in healthy balance with respect to the particular trace element and as we move further to the right there are hidden (or not clinically obvious) signs of toxicity. Later, frank toxicity occurs and in rare cases death can follow. The object of our dietary intake throughout life must clearly be to keep within the centre 'healthy' section at all stages of growth and development.

TOXIC METALS

Certain toxic metals and in particular lead, cadmium and aluminium, are important because they act as 'anti-trace elements'.

Lead has been known for centuries to be toxic and it is now known that it affects trace element metabolism at levels way below those which cause classical lead poisoning. The main sources of lead pollution are petrol exhaust, coal burning, dust and dirt, leaded house paint, drinking water that has been in lead pipes, some canned foods, vegetables grown by roadsides, milk from cows grazed on polluted pastures, and many other lesser sources. Because lead inhibits zinc-dependent enzymes, and there are least 100 of these in the body, the potential ill-effects are legion. This is exceptionally important because zinc deficiency is already so commonplace in the population generally.

There are several nutritional protective factors that can help prevent the ill-effects of lead. These include vitamin C, zinc, calcium, magnesium, iron, vitamin D, chromium, vitamin E and selenium, and proteins and amino acids.

Aluminium is widely dispersed in our environment and is a real potential hazard because it permeates foods cooked in aluminium cookware. It is also commonly used in household and industrial utensils, packaging materials, cans, and so on. Aluminium salts are added to table salt to prevent it from clogging; to antacids for indigestion; and are also found in deodorants and anti-perspirants. Clearly we are all at some risk of aluminium toxicity.

Most of these environmental sources of aluminium can be avoided with some thought and care and such changes are probably worthwhile in the interests of preserving the balance of one's trace elements.

Cadmium is present in rain water and in water that has lain in galvanized iron tanks. Soft water also dissolves out zinc and cadmium which makes it vital to flush out water from pipes before drinking it early in the morning. Cadmium exerts its negative effects by displacing zinc from important enzymes thus making them inactive. Vitamin C, iron and zinc all protect against cadmium toxicity. Cigarette smokers are particularly at risk from cadmium toxicity because not only do cigarettes yield cadmium into the smoker's lungs but smoking lowers vitamin C, a proven protective against this toxic metal.

In general then it makes sense to minimize the effects of toxic metals. This can be done as follows:

● Avoid exposure at work or at home.
● Stop smoking.
● Get rid of your aluminium cooking pots.
● Eat plenty of fibre and nutrient-rich vegetables and fruits.
● Avoid fruit and vegetables on display outside greengrocers' shops if they are on a busy road (or be sure to wash them well).
● Correct any nutritional deficiencies by improving your diet.

Figure 1. The effects of too little or too much of a trace element.

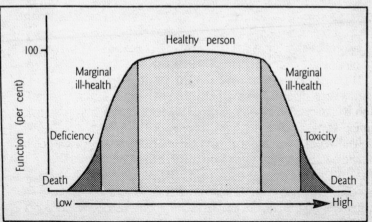

CHAPTER TWO

THE SOURCES OF TRACE ELEMENTS

All trace elements originally come from the soil. They go from there into the water supply, plants and animals, all of which we then consume as food and drink. Table 1 shows how much of various trace elements we need and how much we get.

Table 1. Body content, daily requirements and daily intakes of trace elements in adults (approximate values in mg)*

Element	Body content	Daily requirements	Dietary intake	% absorbed from diet
Silicon	18000	3	20	1
Iron	4200	10	13	7
Fluorine	2600	1	0.3	85
Zinc	2300	3	13	20
Copper	75	2	5	35
Vanadium	25	0.003	2	5
Iodine	20	0.2	0.2	100
Selenium	20	?	0.1	60
Tin	17	3	3	1
Manganese	15	2.5	4	3
Nickel	10	0.02	0.4	5
Molybdenum	9	0.1	0.2	50
Chromium	6	0.2	0.1	10
Cobalt	1.5	0.00004	0.3	80
Calcium	10^6	800	1000	30
Magnesium	19000	350	300	35

* Data taken from various sources and published by the World Health Organisation in WHO Chronicle, 32: 1978.

WATER AS A SOURCE OF TRACE ELEMENTS

For many years water was thought to be unimportant as a source of trace elements but this has now been disproven. Not only does the average person take in about 2 litres of water a day, 60 per cent of which is tap water, but the chemical composition of the food we eat is greatly affected by the chemical composition of the water used to process, prepare and cook it. Food cooked in soft water loses trace elements and that cooked in hard water gains them.

Because we all consume so much water in various forms, the intake of trace elements present at even the tiniest levels can be appreciable. Also, trace elements and other minerals in water are in a particularly absorbable form so once again it would be foolish to ignore them. Normal tap water can provide more than 10 per cent of a person's requirements for calcium, copper, fluorine, iron, lithium, magnesium and zinc and whilst this isn't essential to those who have an adequate dietary intake, it certainly can be to those who have marginal deficiencies and it could make all the difference between life-long optimal or sub-optimal states of health.

Some beneficial trace elements found in water

Lithium is a mood stabilizer which is used in the treatment of depression, and studies have found that populations whose drinking water naturally contains sufficient amounts of the element are less aggressive and less competitive than others. For example, studies in Texas found lower mortality rates from heart attacks, a smaller number of admissions for mental disorders and a lower frequency of violent behaviour such as homicides and suicides in certain areas that differed from neighbouring ones only in the amount of lithium in the drinking water. Water in the low-rate areas contained much more lithium than in the high-rate areas. The low prevalence of coronary heart disease and gastro-duodenal ulcers and the quiet ways of the Pima Indians are thought to be linked to the exceptionally high lithium content of their water supplies, which contain 50 times the average US tap water content of lithium.

Chromium is now known to play an essential role in glucose metabolism (see page 00) and a study in Jordan showed a link between a lack of chromium in the drinking water and juvenile diabetes. The study looked at two Jordanian villages similar in every way but for their water supply. When chromium chloride was given to the children in the low-chromium water village juvenile diabetes quickly disappeared.

Chromium has also been found to be protective against atherosclerosis (hardening of the arteries) in animals. In Man too, chromium in the drinking water may protect to some extent against coronary heart disease. In the eastern part of Finland where there is a very high rate of coronary heart disease there is only a third as much chromium in the drinking water as there is in the western part where coronary heart disease is much less common.

Fluorine hardly needs to be 'sold' in its protective role against dental caries. It's difficult to get enough from food sources (though swallowed toothpaste can be a meaningful source in young children) and 60 per cent of the body's requirements have to come from water. Calcification of the aorta (the main outflow from the heart) is less prevalent in areas where the tap water is rich in fluorine and in Finland lower rates of coronary heart disease have been reported in areas where the drinking water contains higher fluorine and magnesium than elsewhere.

Iodine has been recognized as a cure for goitre since antiquity and recent studies in Greece showed that the drinking water in goitrous areas had one seventy-fifth of the amount of iodine compared with that in non-goitrous areas. Similar studies have proven much the same in Iran. Water can contribute up to 20 per cent of the daily requirements of iodine and in Finland very low water-iodine levels have been linked to an increased risk of suffering from coronary heart disease.

Drinking water is, of course, not a uniform product even within the households of one town, and is certainly not comparable from country to country. Hot, soft water will leach out copper or lead from the pipes in which it is carried and whilst this can be beneficial with copper it can be dangerous with regard to lead.

The World Health Organization has suggested that the indiscriminate softening of water (aimed mainly at removing calcium) should be discouraged on the grounds that it removes trace elements too. Certainly some industrial uses for water require that it be softened and it could be argued that domestic appliances running on hot water would also benefit from having a softened water supply, but for human consumption, hard water is better from a trace element point of view.

SOIL, PLANTS AND ANIMALS—THE BASIS OF OUR FOODS

Important though water is with regard to trace elements it is foods that supply most of our needs.

Soil composition depends mostly on the nature of the rocks from which it comes, but over millions of years (and sometimes over a very much shorter time) the nature and composition of soil can change, often dramatically. Highly leached soils, especially if they were never very rich in trace elements, can easily be too poor to provide a healthy environment for the plants and animals they support. Poorly-drained soils contain far more trace elements than well-drained soils of the same type and the availability of trace elements to plants can be considerably altered by the aeration of the soil, its acidity and by the use of manures and fertilizers. Soils all over the world have been studied for their trace element content and it has been found that certain areas of the USA, for example, have soil that is poor in selenium and/or zinc. In fact the shortage of zinc in the soils of at least 30 states in the US has led to enrichment becoming the norm. Repeated intensive cropping of farmland removes more and more of the trace elements, a situation which is made worse by an imbalanced use of fertilizers. Only recently have farmers started the systematic replacement of these losses, which are almost inevitable with modern 'factory farming'.

Plants provide the food for animals and Man, and their trace element content depends on the type of plant species, the nature of the soil on which they are grown, the climatic conditions during growth and the maturity of the plant. Man's activities such as draining, fertilizing, irrigating, weedkilling and the use of pesticides further alter the trace element content of plants. Although most farmers use nitrogenous fertilizers, phosphorus and potash to replace these losses from the soil, few do much, if anything, to replace the trace elements their crops remove year after year.

Some plants, or even certain parts of particular plants, accumulate especially large amounts of specific trace elements. There are well documented selenium, strontium, aluminium and cobalt 'accumulator' plants. Legumes are usually richer in cobalt, nickel, iron, copper and zinc than cereals or grasses, whereas these latter are usually higher in manganese, molybdenum and silicon.

Work by pioneering agriculturalists and veterinarians in the 1930s led to the first descriptions of the importance of trace elements in animal health. Soon they became aware that far more subtle trace element imbalances were at work in the animal population than was at first apparent and that vastly larger numbers suffered from sub-clinical deficiencies and toxic states. Animals living in the wild roam over a large area and aren't as subject to any imbalances there might be in the soil as are domestic farm animals forced to graze very restricted areas. As a result, animal husbandry is more likely to produce trace element deficiency situations than would be encountered in the wild.

This same principle applies in reverse to Man because, today at least, his food comes from widely dispersed geographical areas. So a trace element deficiency in plants from any one area is likely to be made up by an excess accumulation in plants from another.

Because people weren't obviously suffering from any overt problems in the geographical areas in which animals were experiencing substantial trace element deficiencies, the medical and scientific fraternities were loath to accept that trace element deficiencies could occur in people. It has only very recently been realized that subtle clinical syndromes can be caused by trace element insufficiencies.

FOOD AS A SOURCE OF TRACE ELEMENTS

The vast majority of our trace element intake comes from foods and we have seen how these depend ultimately on the soil on which the original plant food sources were grown. We in the West eat few raw foods, and processing, storage and cooking all take their toll of trace elements. We shall look at each of these in turn.

First, the original trace element content of food varies enormously, some plants being much richer in certain elements than others. This points to the importance of a balanced diet containing a broad spectrum of plant and animal foods.

Most of our foods today are processed somehow or other but the most dramatic losses of trace elements occur during refining. Table 2 shows the percentage of elements lost when certain common foods are refined. The figures speak for themselves and are a matter for considerable concern. Table 3 shows the losses of trace elements from wholewheat flour when it is made into white flour.

Table 2. Trace element losses (%) from foodstuffs due to refining (blank spaces indicate that data are unavailable)*

	Mg	Cr	Mn	Co	Cu	Zn	Mo	Fe	Se
Wheat	80	87	88	50	63	75	48	76	
Rice	83	75	27	38	25	50			
Sugar	99	90	89	88	80	98			75
Oil	99					75			
Butter	94					50			

* Based on SCHROEDER, H. A. *The Trace Elements and Man*. Old Greenwich. Devin-Adair Co. Old Greenwich, Con., USA, 1975, and MASIRONI, R. ET AL., Zinc, copper, cadmium, and chromium in polished and unpolished rice. *Sci. total environ.*, 7: 27-43 (1977).

Table 3. Losses of trace elements when wholewheat flour is refined to make white flour.*

Element	Wholewheat	White	Average % loss
Chromium, ppm	1.75	0.23	87
Cobalt, ppm	0.07-0.2	0.05-0.07	70
Copper, ppm	1.8-6.2	0.62-0.63	70-90
Iron, ppm	18-31	3.5-9.1	81
Magnesium, ppm	0.09-0.12	0.013-0.021	83
Manganese, ppm	24-37	2.1-3.5	91
Molybdenum, ppm	0.3-0.66	0.16-0.39	50
Selenium†	0.04-0.71	0.01-0.63	12-75
Zinc, ppm	21-63	3.9-10.5	83

ppm = parts per million, or ten thousandths of a per cent.
* From SCHROEDER, H. A. *The Trace Elements and Man*. Old Greenwich. Devin-Adair Co, Old Greenwich, Conn., USA.
† The selenium content of wheat varies considerably depending on the soil where the crop grew.

So the reduced trace element content of the original plant (because of repeated cropping on increasingly poor soil) is further reduced by the food processing industry. But this isn't the end.

Freezing also takes its toll as can be seen from Table 4. Freezing isn't a bad way of preserving food by and large, but the blanching that precedes the freezing of vegetables and fruits can remove substantial proportions of their zinc, calcium and manganese. When frozen meat thaws, several trace elements (including iron) are lost in the drips, and the freezing of fish is thought to cause a loss of iodine.

Table 4. Percentage loss of calcium and magnesium in frozen fruits and vegetables*

Fruits	Ca	Mg	Vegetables	Ca	Mg
Apricots	33	12	Asparagus	0	30
Blackberries	56	48	Lima beans	33	38
Blueberries	53	0	Green beans	19	34
Strawberries	39	31	Black peas	7	0
Cherries	22	0	Brussels sprouts	33	9
Peaches	33	40	Corn	57	53
Average % loss	45	28	Green peas	4	31
			Potatoes	0	38
			Spinach	0	23
			Average % loss	17	30

*Data from HANKIN, J. H. ET AL. Contribution of hard water to calcium and magnesium intakes of adults. *J. Am. diet Assoc.*, 56: 212 (1970).

Once in the kitchen the trouble continues. Pressure cooking foods or heating them vigorously removes some trace elements and peeling removes yet more. Peeling potatoes, for example, removes three quarters of their fluorine. Losses are particularly high if the food is cooked in lots of water which is then discarded. The average housewife buys quite a lot of trace elements but then throws them away. The outer leaves of vegetables are rich in minerals yet are discarded and last of all we stew food for a long time in lots of water and then throw the rich water away instead of using it. Unfortunately, such dietary and food preparation habits are passed on in families so the children of a trace element-deficient family continue to deprive their children in the same way their parents did.

Assuming we do get a nutritious, balanced diet, fairly rich in trace elements, what happens once we eat it?

Knowledge about the absorption mechanisms of the trace elements and what controls them is still pretty scanty except for zinc, iodine and iron which have been widely studied. What is known is that uptake is influenced by the body's need for the element. So, for example, someone who is iron-deficient will absorb double the iron of a person whose body's iron stores are full. The uptake of one trace element also affects and is affected by the uptake of others. Medication with iron, for example, can adversely affect the absorption of copper, and zinc depresses copper absorption and vice versa. Cobalt and iron compete for absorption mechanisms in the intestine and many other interactions are known to affect the absorption of the trace elements that are there. Zinc and iron absorption are substantially reduced by the intake of a high-fibre diet because the phytic acid contained in cereal-based foods binds these elements which are then lost in the stools. This can be a very important source of loss if the diet is only marginally supplied with trace elements and is high in fibre. It's also interesting that zinc and iron absorption are inhibited especially by tea and to a lesser extent by coffee drinking. We also lose trace elements in the urine and urine volumes go up when we drink tea or coffee because they have an effect on the kidneys that makes them produce more urine than the volume of tea or coffee actually drunk.

In general, animal foodstuffs have a higher content and greater availability of a large amount of trace elements than do plant foodstuffs. Oysters and other seafoods appear to be particularly rich in both the essential and the so-called toxic elements.

Breast milk, a balanced and rich source of trace elements (if the mother is eating a balanced diet) has been replaced as the main food source for their babies by many mothers with a manufactured product of cows' milk—baby formula—the trace element content of which often differs markedly in different products, some of which are extremely low in individual essential elements and are frequently less available to the baby than the trace elements in breast milk. The implications of this are far reaching but we cannot go into them here.

Once in the intestine, only a tiny proportion of most of the trace elements present in food is absorbed. Chromium is a good example of this. Regardless of the dose or quantity of chromium in an individual, absorption amounts to 1 per cent or less if chromium is present in the diet in the trivalent form; when it is present as a complex known as the 'glucose tolerance factor' absorption is good (see page 41). Egg yolk is rich in chromium but in a form which is of low nutritional value. Table 1 summarized the daily requirements for the trace elements, the total body content, dietary intake and the percentage that is absorbed from the diet. A concept of recommended daily requirements is an attractive one in theory but is very difficult to work out in practice, and various countries around the world have very different recommended 'normal' intakes. As we have seen, it's almost pointless to define such norms if only because no one can really know how much he or she is taking in the form of foods, given the considerable variations in food content and absorption that have been mentioned. Even if trace elements were taken as food supplements in regulated doses one couldn't be sure exactly how much was being absorbed by any one individual, and his uptake of them will vary anyway according to his state of health, stress, age, drug intake and many other factors. It is possible though, by measuring how much of each trace element is lost from the body in all forms, to arrive at a sensible figure for the body's daily needs because presumably that same amount has to be replaced if the person is not to become deficient in that element. However, simply to give the same amount in the diet is clearly not sensible, given that we know that such a small proportion of all dietary sources of trace elements ends up being absorbed. The dilemma then in recommending 'ideal' daily doses lies in knowing how large a multiplication factor to allow in order to compensate for very variable absorption rates.

But it's not just how much of a particular trace element one consumes that's important; it also matters in what form it's taken. Presumably these forms sort themselves out in a natural, healthy, balanced diet, but when it comes to giving trace element supplements the story is more complex because pure trace elements themselves in the form of simple inorganic salts are sometimes poorly absorbed and need to be complexed in some way to help things along. Some have been grown into yeast (selenium is a good example of this); others chelated, as in nature, with amino acids; and yet others combined with orotic acid (a B-vitamin). All of these give provably better absorption of trace elements than when using the pure substances alone.

SOME READILY-AVAILABLE SOURCES OF ESSENTIAL TRACE ELEMENTS

Chromium
Beef, beer, molasses, brewer's yeast, grape juice, offal, whole grains, shellfish, liver, kidney.

Cobalt
Meats, fish, dairy foods, eggs, liver, kidney.

Copper
Liver, kidney, shellfish, nuts, stone fruits, whole grains, legume seeds, oysters, green vegetables, beef extract.

Fluorine
Tea, seafood, sea salt.

Iodine
Black pudding, offal, game, shellfish, soya beans, dried apricots, whole grains, sardines, molasses, beef, lamb, dark green vegetables, wholemeal bread.

Manganese
Nuts, whole grains, legume seeds, fruits, liver and kidney, spices, tea, green leafy vegetables.

Molybdenum
Widespread in many foods. Content varies greatly with soil's molybdenum content. Whole grains, wheat germ, liver, lima beans, soya beans, sunflower seeds.

Selenium
Seafood, meat, seaweed, brewer's yeast, eggs, garlic.

Zinc
Seafood, meat, whole grains, nuts, pulses, kidney, rice.

CHAPTER THREE

TRACE ELEMENTS IN SPECIAL SITUATIONS

PREGNANCY

It is well known that a growing baby inside its mother's uterus requires substantial amounts of nutrients of all kinds if it is to grow optimally. Information is scanty about the trace element needs of the foetus but studies have been done into the copper, zinc and iron needs before birth. The practice of giving high doses of iron during pregnancy is being questioned, if only because it inhibits zinc absorption and possibly that of other trace elements. Certainly sufficient trace elements must be available if the baby is to be healthy and there is good evidence from animal research that a deficiency of certain specific trace elements can produce abnormal foetuses. The problem of supplementing pregnant women with trace elements remains but there is at least some evidence that small doses (5-10mg/day) of zinc are useful for certain women.

Some women feel 'down' after pregnancy—not depressed but generally 'unwell'. In some of these an imbalance of zinc to copper, or a deficiency of magnesium or zinc alone seem to be the problem.

BABY FEEDING

There is probably no other time in our lives when we need a healthy diet more than in the first year when our organs (and especially the brain) are growing at their fastest ever. Yet in spite of this fact being widely appreciated by the medical profession and the public alike few women choose to breast-feed for even the suggested four month minimum and most have stopped well before this.

There is now no doubt at all that breast-feeding is the best way to nourish a baby. It also has many other benefits but they aren't within the scope of this book. Yet even knowing this, the medical and para-medical professions still often give the impression that cows' milk (meant to nourish calves) is as good as human milk for human babies. Whilst it is undoubtedly true that baby milk formula is a modified form of cows' milk which, in its currently available form, brings it tolerably close to human milk in its main nutritional constituents, many of the vital constituents of breast milk (some of them living) that are known to be essential for human growth and health are either totally absent from formula or are present in different concentrations from those in breast milk.

A study in Tasmania in 1974 found that the concentration of trace elements in baby formulae varied considerably from feed to feed and from the manufacturers' specifications. Given that no one knows exactly how many trace elements a baby needs to be healthy and grow properly, the formula manufacturers have set themselves an impossible task. It is well known that the composition of breast milk changes as lactation progresses and even within any one feed. Could there be a reason for this which could not be catered for by giving a manufactured formula milk of constant composition? Studies over the years have suggested that breast milk was low in certain trace elements but an increasing understanding of the subject suggests that there's probably a very good reason for this. Also, methods of measuring certain trace elements have not always been accurate enough to be able to be sure what really is there and on other occasions the wrong things have been measured. A good example of this was to say that breast milk was low in copper. However, copper is better absorbed from breast milk than from cows' milk formula (iron too is absorbed twice as readily from breast milk as it is from cows' milk formula) so the actual amount of available copper is much higher than would at first appear. Also, evidence in rats shows that the ratio of zinc to copper in cows' milk formula is disadvantageous to the absorption of copper—so once again the facts speak for themselves.

The factors that influence the trace element composition of human milk are poorly understood but they probably depend to some extent on the mother's diet. Having said this, simply giving a lactating woman more of a particular trace element doesn't immediately raise the amount of it appearing in her milk. Perhaps some goes into her body stores or it could be that at that phase of lactation the milk shouldn't contain that particular trace element anyway. The guideline for breast-feeding mothers must be to eat a nutritious, balanced diet rich in foods likely to contain trace elements because it is well recognized that the drain of trace elements into breast milk (and thence to the baby) is considerable during breast-feeding. Many mothers are already trace element deficient (as judged by currently accepted norms) the day they start to breast-feed and so need to increase their food sources of trace elements—sometimes quite substantially (see page 24).

THE GROWING YEARS

During childhood and adolescence there is an increased need for many of the trace elements because they are essential for growth. Millions of children the world over are getting too few either because of frank malnutrition (which is the case for two thirds of the world's children) or because their food consists of highly-refined, processed or 'junk' food (the main problem for the other third). There's little doubt that many children today will remain short of trace elements unless their parents make a conscious effort to give them natural, unrefined foods or a supplement. This danger is especially high in large families and those on a low income.

Zinc deficiency is very common in childhood and results in sleep disturbances, poor growth, and behaviour and learning problems.

SLIMMING

We live in a society which is obsessed with slimming—or rather with obesity. There is no doubt that obesity kills people unnecessarily young and adversely affects the lives of others by producing diseases not seen in the slim, but the way that millions of women especially choose to slim can seriously hazard their trace element intake. Many cranky diets and even some balanced slimming diets simply contain so little of any food substances that by definition there are too few trace elements. After all, if you are eating almost nothing, no matter how nutritious it is, you won't get much out of it. Certain slimming diets are actually harmful and some have even caused deaths because of the dramatic reduction in trace element intake (liquid protein diets causing copper deficiency are an example). It makes sense to eat a reasonably balanced diet when slimming and to shy completely away from single food 'fad' diets because they cannot possibly provide all that the body needs. It would be a reasonable safe-guard to take multi-vitamin and multi-trace element supplements too for the same reason.

INFECTIONS

Infections alter the body's metabolism of iron, zinc and copper and these are known to be of major importance in combating infection. Changes also occur in manganese, cobalt, gallium, iodine and chromium levels in people with infections but whether these changes are the cause or the effect isn't known. The total body balance of iron and copper remains much the same during an infection but most studies show that zinc levels fall. Zinc is taken up by the liver and copper is released by it. Trace element metabolism is profoundly affected by infection and the body's distribution of the elements can change considerably. Certain trace elements accumulate at the site of the infection and high fevers produced by infections alter the body's normal transport mechanisms of trace elements.

No one knows why these trace element changes occur but they are probably part of a sort of defence mobilization system. What is certain is that people with low levels of iron, zinc, copper and magnesium are more susceptible to infections and that often their infections are more serious than they should be.

DRUGS

As trace elements are so intimately tied up with the very basis of metabolism itself, it is hardly surprising that foreign chemicals that alter the body's metabolism generally have an effect on trace element metabolism in particular. Several studies have also found that the dietary levels of zinc, magnesium, iron, copper and calcium alter the rate of drug metabolism—so the story is a two-way one. Unfortunately, knowledge about the effects of trace elements on the action of most drugs and vice versa is very scanty and a lot of research still needs to be done. The fact that many drugs are metabolized and detoxified in the liver, which is the body's main store of trace elements, cannot be ignored and we don't yet know the effects of low liver stores of particular trace elements on the metabolism of individual drugs. With so many people taking drugs of one kind or another (even if it's only nicotine in cigarettes) more research is needed to see what effects they are having on trace element metabolism and vice versa.

The anti-inflammatory drug prednisolone is known to reduce potassium, magnesium and zinc; penicillamine, used in arthritis, reduces zinc and

Table 5 Groups that are at special risk of trace element deficiency and their most likely shortages.

	Zinc	Chromium	Iron	Manganese
Alcoholics	●	●		
Diabetics	●	●		
Vegetarians	●		●	
Heavy tea drinkers	●		●	
Pregnant women	●		●	
Lactating women	●			
Refined carbohydrate eaters	●	●		●
Anyone with malabsorption	●	●	●	●

copper; certain 'water tablets' increase the amount of magnesium and zinc put out in the urine; certain anti-epilepsy drugs can increase copper and reduce zinc levels (the contraceptive Pill does the same); and alcohol increases body losses of zinc, chromium, magnesium and potassium and can actually cause deficiencies of these minerals.

OLD AGE

The old, suffering as they sometimes do from nutritional problems generally, are more likely than most to be short of trace elements. The elderly often find it difficult to get out to the shops and so tend to buy convenience foods with a long shelf life, many of which are low in trace elements. Some also eat very little of anything at all (like slimmers) and those who have lost all their natural teeth have to choose foods that they can eat with dentures. All of this makes at least some of the elderly more susceptible to trace element deficiencies. Most would probably benefit from vitamin and trace element supplements. Many of the elderly are also on medication which often seems to produce more ill-effects in them than in younger people. Could it be that their poor diet, low in trace elements, doesn't supply enough of these vital substances to enable them to metabolize drugs normally? Research continues, but in the meantime it makes sense to do everything possible to bring an old person's intake of trace elements up to normal, however this is achieved. Degenerative changes in the body's vital organs such as the liver and the kidneys also alter the body's ability to handle and excrete trace elements—another reason for the elderly being at greater risk from trace element imbalance.

CHAPTER FOUR

TRACE ELEMENTS AND ILL HEALTH

We shall look at the specific action of each trace element and its effects in too high or too low a level in Chapter 6, but here let's look at some more general principles.

Although animals can, and do, suffer very real problems from several well-proven trace element deficiencies, such gross examples are rarely seen in humans. Longstanding marginal deficiencies are, however, very common indeed. Unfortunately, many such abnormalities in Man aren't obviously related to a disease and so tend to have been ignored or even scorned. Things are now set to change however because evidence is accumulating all over the world to prove how wrong these views are. Given that so many trace elements are crucial to the functioning of enzyme systems it wouldn't be surprising to find that there was a trace element problem that was central to many chronic diseases.

Although the subject is vast and the research data prolific, let's just look at a few common conditions that we know to be affected by changes in the states of various trace elements.

Loss of appetite is a common symptom of a deficiency of many, if not most, trace elements but especially of zinc and cobalt.

Cancer, it has been suggested, is linked to a deficiency of selenium (see page 56).

Cardiovascular disease. Suggestions that the risks of this are enhanced by chromium, copper and selenium deficiencies are now being carefully evaluated. Excess lead and cadmium can cause heart disease. But as with cancer, there are undoubtedly many other variables involved.

Dental caries is preventable to a great extent by taking fluoride, yet there are 43 other known constituents of developing human tooth enamel.

Carbohydrate metabolism is now known to need chromium, and old people who can't handle glucose properly can be helped by taking chromium supplements. People with diabetes tend to lose quite a lot of potassium, magnesium, chromium and zinc in their urine and as a result their requirements for these elements increase.

Abnormalities in foetal development have been produced in experimental animals by diets deficient in manganese, magnesium, zinc, chromium and several other trace elements. Deficiencies of any of these elements can produce abnormal or stillborn offspring (as can lead or cadmium excess). Animal studies have shown especially that zinc deprivation during pregnancy results in a weak immune system in their offspring and that this weakness takes three generations to be rectified. The same appears to occur with magnesium.

Infections, increasingly, are realized to be more likely in trace element-deficient people. Some trace elements are necessary for the functioning of the immune system that fights infection. Zinc and iron are especially valuable in this context.

Skin (and hair and nail) condition is sensitive to a deficiency of certain trace elements. Deficiencies of iodine and zinc are especially likely to produce skin problems. In Man 20 per cent of body zinc is in the skin. In juvenile diabetics the chromium content of the hair is 50 per cent lower than that of normal children.

Wound and burn healing is greatly improved by zinc.

Fertility is undoubtedly affected by trace element deficiencies: notable in this area are shortages of iodine and zinc. Just how big a role trace element deficiencies play in human infertility isn't yet known but we do know that zinc is of paramount importance in the production of sperms and that zinc-deficient men have a low sperm count with increased numbers of abnormal forms. The same applies to selenium deficiency. Mercury, lead and cadmium excesses also cause an increased number of abnormal sperms and thus reduce fertility. People who are extremely zinc-deficient (or indeed who are very low in many other trace elements) have a decreased sex drive which in turn makes them less likely to produce children.

Skeletal abnormalities occur with deficiences of copper, zinc and manganese and with fluorine and molybdenum toxicities.

Special senses. Taste is impaired or lost with zinc deficiency, as is the sense of smell. It is also thought that night blindness can be caused by zinc deficiency.

Thyroid disorders due to a lack of iodine are said to affect 200 million people, mainly in iodine-deficient areas of the world.

Mental function is profoundly affected by imbalances of zinc, manganese, magnesium, calcium and copper. This can produce depression, insomnia, poor concentration and other problems all of which can disappear when the imbalances are corrected.

CHAPTER FIVE

HOW TO GET ENOUGH TRACE ELEMENTS FROM YOUR DIET

1. Eat a balanced, nutritious diet containing as wide a variety of foods as you reasonably can. This advice is especially important for children, adolescents, the pregnant and breast-feeding, and the elderly.
2. Eat fresh foods in season whenever possible.
3. Keep away from 'cranky' diets, especially for slimming.
4. Eat whole (unrefined and unprocessed) foods whenever possible.
5. Eat as much of the outer leaves and parts of vegetables as is reasonable but be sure to wash fruit and vegetables purchased from open displays at the roadside.
6. Peel fruit and vegetables as little as possible to preserve the trace elements stored immediately under the skin.
7. Don't leave fruit or vegetables soaking in water before cooking.
8. Never leave opened cans with food still in them—trace elements can be rendered unavailable to the body by the action of the components of the tin dissolved off by the acids in foods in the presence of air.
9. Cook foods in the least amount of fluid you can and then use the liquid for sauces, soups and casseroles.
10. Cook food quickly for a minimum of time.
11. Avoid pressure cooking if possible—steam-heat under pressure removes many valuable trace elements from foods.
12. Take a trace element supplement if you are proven to be short of a particular element; if you are unable to eat a healthy, balanced diet as outlined above; or if you are in one of the groups likely to be vulnerable to a deficiency of these elements (see (1) above). The tolerance to many trace elements is reasonably high and you are very unlikely to take too much if you stick to the instructions of a reputable manufacturer who is himself guided by the widely accepted dosage levels.

If you do take a trace element supplement either as a food or as a 'medication' don't expect immediate results if you are suffering from a deficiency. Sometimes the results are dramatic if the deficiency is severe but this is uncommon and results will usually take weeks or months to become apparent. Remember too to take commercially prepared supplements in between meals rather than with food as this increases the amount that is absorbed from them.

Most important though is to be sure that you report to your doctor any worsening of your symptoms or a failure to improve, because it could be that what you or he is treating is something else and not the trace element deficiency you or he thought.

Many people today, however hard they try and however healthily they eat, are probably consuming too few vitamins and trace elements, especially during periods of growth, during pregnancy and breast-feeding, and in old age. It's very difficult with today's processed foods to be sure that one is getting a reasonable balance of trace elements and supplementation does no known harm and could do a lot of good. Even so-called 'natural' health foods are often grown on soils poor in trace elements, so it's difficult to approach what our ancestors would have eaten even a few hundred years ago, let alone thousands of years ago. Environmental pollution too contaminates our air, soil and food and disturbs the natural balances of trace elements still further by replacing helpful and useful elements with harmful, toxic ones. All of this makes the job of maintaining a healthy trace element balance more uncertain than ever. Just how many of our modern diseases and ailments are the result of such an imbalance is impossible to say but it would be surprising if they did not play an important part, involved as trace elements are at the very heart of life itself.

HOW DO I KNOW IF I AM SHORT OF A PARTICULAR TRACE ELEMENT?

The simple answer is that you probably won't know unless, of course, you are suffering from an obvious clinical deficiency syndrome such as those outlined in Chapter 6. The vast majority of trace element deficiencies produce subclinical (not obvious) problems—many of which are not yet fully recognized or understood. As doctors become more aware of the early signs of trace element deficiencies they'll be better able to pick up more and more of them and to predict those people likely to find themselves in 'at risk' situations and so prevent problems occurring at all.

There is still considerable debate as to how to assess the body's trace element status and this is hardly surprising because at any one time some trace elements are being absorbed (are in the intestine as food); others are in transit to their stores or target organs where they act (and are measurable in the blood); while others are actually in these stores and target organs themselves. The study of urine, blood, stools, hair and nails all yield some information but it is very difficult to interpret because the body's natural control mechanisms tend to keep the supply to the target organs as constant as possible whatever the state of the body's stores of the particular trace element under consideration. So, for example, one could find that the blood level of a particular element is normal yet the body as a whole could be short of it as it calls on the last of its stores to keep going effectively.

If as a result of reading this book you think you might have a trace element deficiency, discuss it with your doctor.

One of the reasons for the increasing interest in trace elements is that over the last 25 years our ability to measure substances present in such minute quantities has leaped forward in giant steps. Today, with sophisticated equipment, trace elements present at the parts per billion level can be measured in almost any body fluid or tissue. However, such methods are time-consuming and fairly costly so the medical profession has been looking around to find a way of screening people for gross abnormalities in trace elements, abnormalities which could then be investigated in more detail, if required. On the grounds of public acceptability and cost all the highly sophisticated measuring methods are ruled out for screening. This leaves one increasingly popular method—hair analysis.

HAIR MINERAL ANALYSIS

Until the last 10 years or so interest in analysing the content of human hair was confined almost entirely to its use in forensic medicine when it was often helpful in 'proving' that someone had been poisoned. The procedure has also been useful in understanding more about historical figures because hair is durable and can give interesting insights into people's health when they were alive. Napoleon's hair has, for example, been found to be rich in arsenic.

Today, hair analysis plays an increasingly important role in the story of environmental pollution and mineral (especially trace element) nutrition. Some 55 elements have been identified in human hair, their concentrations ranging from a few parts per billion to about 4.5 per cent by weight.

There are several reasons why hair analysis has become so popular, especially in the USA. First, although blood plasma or serum is the most respected and established source of information on the body's biochemical status, the extremely low concentrations of the trace elements in blood make it difficult to measure them accurately. Second, although many trace elements can be accurately measured in the blood, there is no certainty that what one is measuring reflects the body's true trace element status. In fact, research suggests that blood measurements are dependent upon recent dietary intake rather than the 'whole body' picture. Of course, other body tissues could be used for the measurement of trace elements, and urine, saliva and nail clippings have all been examined in this context.

With an increasing interest in trace elements both within and outside the medical profession it's not surprising that hair analysis has caught on the way it has. Collection of the sample is simple; it can be done by the patient himself (unlike blood-taking); it causes no pain or damage; and the sample so obtained can be transported easily. Trace element concentrations in the hair are often fairly high, thus making the laboratory work easier (and so more accurate) and probably most important of all, hair, because it grows so slowly, can give an historic picture over several months or even years as to what was happening at the time. Also, blood levels of trace elements tend to fluctuate a lot according to dietary intake, whereas hair levels 'smooth out' these hour-by-hour or day-by-day variations and so give a more accurate overall picture of the person's trace element status over a period of time.

All of these advantages have been rightly claimed by laboratories offering hair analysis, but there is reason for caution too. First, the hair, having obviously been a part of the body for a long time, may well have picked up traces of elements from the environment, traces which have little or nothing to do with the person's body level of that element. This is especially true for industrial pollutants and poisons. It is possible that even very good laboratory washing of the sample will not completely remove such surface contamination and this causes concern to anyone working in this area. This disadvantage becomes even more important when one realizes that people put things onto their hair in the form of hair dressings, shampoos, perms, setting lotions and so on. Many of these contain trace elements. For example, some shampoos contain selenium and others zinc.

Even if the specimen to be analysed is clean (in scientific terms) when the analysis is done there are other variables that have to be taken into account. The colour of the hair can have an effect on its trace element content. For example, manganese concentrations are higher in black hair than in white. The position on the scalp also influences trace element concentrations within any one individual. Finally the interpretation of the results rests on the assumption of normal hair growth. At any one time scalp hairs are in a resting stage or a growth stage. If the analysis was of only a small number of hairs the chance selection of large numbers of resting hairs could make the information atypical. On the other hand hair trace element levels can be very high if the person is starving and so limiting his hair growth—zinc being the best example. In this case we see an elevated hair level of zinc in a person who is in fact zinc-deficient.

So it is clear that hair analysis, however appealing, can't be relied on to give final answers to a person's trace element status. It can, however, be a useful survey method to pick out those who need further in-depth study and this is a perfectly valid use. However, any hair analysis result must be interpreted with caution and with a full knowledge of the person and his lifestyle. Details of the use of hair preparations and shampoos, etc, are essential as is a knowledge of the drugs the person is taking. Hair perming, highlighting and bleaching can produce a calcium, copper and zinc picture that is meaningless and the metabolism of several trace elements is altered if a woman is taking the contraceptive pill. The person's diet must be known, especially if it is an unusual one and, as we have seen, hair colour is a variable worth considering. Hair length, the sex of the individual, his age, and for certain elements even the time of year, have also to be known if the analysis is to be sensibly interpreted. If all of these are taken into account, hair analysis is indeed a useful tool and can suggest further tests that could be done to elucidate the true trace element position before starting treatment.

Because readers may well end up sending a hair sample off for analysis to a commercial laboratory here are some guidelines for the collection of hair.

The hair should be taken from as near the scalp as possible and using the method detailed here there should be no unsightly hair loss. Hair taken too far from the scalp can cause falsely high levels of calcium, magnesium, zinc and copper to be reported.

1.   Make a parting across the back of the head along a line running from the top of one ear to the top of the other.
2.   Fold the hair up from this point.
3.   Below this point, gather a lock of hair together and cut it as close to the scalp as possible.
4.   If the hair is longer than 6–8cm cut off the part further most from the head and discard it and send off the 6–8cm nearest to the scalp to the laboratory.
5.   Place the sample in a clean envelope (about 2 tablespoonsful are usually enough).

Once the analysis has been done, most commercial laboratories give some kind of interpretation of the results and make suggestions as to the dietary changes that would affect the situation advantageously. If you are in any doubt see your doctor who will have blood or other estimations done if he is at all concerned. Of course ideally you should have the procedure carried out under the supervision of a suitably trained doctor who can help you interpret the results, but this is often not possible.

CHAPTER SIX

THE TEN ESSENTIAL TRACE ELEMENTS

CHROMIUM

The biological significance of this trace element has only recently been recognized but now that it has been there are signs that many people are short of it. Chromium is physiologically active in the body in only one inorganic form (the trivalent form). This inorganic (non-living) type of chromium is very inactive in the body compared with another chromium-containing compound, the organic complex called the glucose tolerance factor (GTF). It appears that animals have only a limited ability to produce it themselves and so need external sources. GTF is the only known form in which chromium can cross the placenta. When trivalent chromium is given orally less than 1 per cent is absorbed.

Chromium's main function is to help insulin to control the body's sugar levels. Experiments with animals have found that glucose (sugar) metabolism is quickly impaired if they are fed diets poor in chromium and that giving the element soon returns the situation to normal. Because research found that chromium-deficient animals developed diabetes-like symptoms, it seemed natural to ask whether a similar mechanism could be at fault in human diabetes. Several reports have suggested that giving chromium has had beneficial effects on diabetics, and in one study 4 out of 6 maturity-onset diabetics improved with a dose of 250 micrograms of chromium a day. Studies of poorly nourished children in Jordan, Turkey and Nigeria found that they grew faster when given extra chromium. In spite of this circumstantial evidence there is no definite evidence to suggest that diabetes is caused by a deficiency of chromium, and it is certain that many diabetics will not find their condition improved simply by taking chromium.

Heart disease may be linked to chromium deficiency but the evidence is patchy. Interest in this area is based on three main findings. First, chromium-deficient rats have very high blood cholesterol levels and this is known to predispose to a clogging up of the arteries; second, some human subjects have had their blood cholesterol levels reduced after taking chromium supplements; and third, western people have lower blood chromium levels than do others living in low-heart disease areas of the world. People living in non-westernized areas have high body chromium stores which reduce when they emigrate to the West.

In one study, those dying of coronary heart disease were found to have almost no chromium in their aortas where those dying of accidents and other diseases had plenty. Studies in both animals and humans suggest that chromium deficiency combined with excessive sugar intake could be an important nutritional factor in heart disease. Chromium deficiency tends to decrease the liver's uptake of cholesterol and fatty acids and this could favour the deposition and accumulation of the fats in the arteries.

Signs and symptoms of deficiency

There are none reported at present and certainly diabetes and heart disease cannot be said to be caused simply by chromium deficiency—there are undoubtedly many other factors involved. The groups of people most likely to become deficient are the pregnant; those diabetics who are insulin-dependent (who lose chromium in the urine); slimmers; and those living in areas where the concentration of chromium is low in the soil. People on a very refined diet almost certainly become chromium, manganese and zinc deficient. Three pointers to the necessity of chromium in Man are an impaired ability of the body to handle sugar—which is improved with an increased chromium intake; a measurably low level of chromium in the hair of some diabetic children; and a low concentration of chromium in the urine.

Apart from those mentioned above (slimmers, the elderly, insulin-dependent diabetics, the pregnant and those living in low-chromium soil areas), the largest group of people likely to be short of this element world-wide are the severely malnourished in the developing countries. This means that chromium deficiency could be a very common problem indeed world-wide.

How to get enough chromium

Unfortunately, the refining of foods removes a very substantial part of their chromium. Blackstrap molasses, honey and raw sugar are rich in chromium but white sugar has almost none. This is especially unfortunate since chromium is needed if the body is to handle sugar effectively, as we have seen. White bread contains only one third of the chromium of the original whole wheat and this, of course, goes for anything made from white flour.

The food richest in chromium is brewer's yeast but whole-grain breads, nuts, shellfish, liver, kidneys, grape juice, beef, beer and molasses are also rich sources.

As with many other trace elements, absorption is very poor, especially from tablets. Overall only about 3 per cent of the chromium in our food is absorbed so with our relatively chromium-deficient diet there isn't much of a safety margin.

The recommended daily intake of chromium varies from 5–100 micrograms a day. Given that the body needs to absorb about 10 micrograms a day and that only 3 per cent is absorbed, perhaps the amount we consume should be even higher than 100 micrograms.

COBALT

Cobalt is probably unique among the trace elements in that it is physiologically active in Man mainly when supplied in one specific form—cyanocobalamin or vitamin B_{12}. So to all intents and purposes the study of cobalt in Man becomes the study of vitamin B_{12}. All ruminant animals (in contrast to Man with his single stomach) use dietary cobalt itself, which is converted into vitamin B_{12} in their stomachs. Man depends largely on these animals for his supply of vitamin B_{12} and so is at the end of the cobalt food chain.

The discovery, in the 1930s, that cobalt was essential to sheep and cattle was the foundation stone of the modern story and understanding of trace elements in general. This led to the concept of low soil trace element content, and slowly doctors began to wonder whether humans could be similarly affected. It wasn't until 1948 though that cobalt was found to be an essential part of the vitamin B_{12} molecule. Even with increasing knowledge on the subject much is still ill-understood. For example, some non-B_{12} cobalt is absorbed by the body from food yet what it does is a mystery. Some animal work suggests that cobalt is needed to make thyroid hormones.

Signs and symptoms of deficiency

No signs of a deficiency of cobalt itself are recognized, only signs of vitamin B_{12} deficiency. A lack of this vitamin produces anaemia (pernicious anaemia), muscular weakness, gastro-intestinal disturbances and eventually disease of the nervous tissue. It used to be fatal before the discovery of vitamin B_{12}.

How to get enough

Foods rich in vitamin B_{12} (and so cobalt), are liver, kidney, muscle meats, milk, eggs, cheese and fish. Yeast and soya beans are the main sources of B_{12} acceptable to vegetarians and vegans and some fermented foods also contain a little.

The body controls the amount of B_{12} it absorbs and natural overdoses are unlikely. No cobalt supplements are available commercially for human use so again overdose is unlikely. However, an overdose of cobalt can produce illness. In 1966 it was discovered that very heavy beer drinkers developed a strange type of heart muscle condition which led to heart failure. This was thought to be caused by the cobalt added to preserve the frothy 'head' of the beer. This practice of adding cobalt is no longer acceptable, and anyway it is thought that the excessive intake of cobalt has to be accompanied by a poor protein intake in order to produce these dramatic effects on the heart. Apart from this 'beer drinkers' cardiomyopathy' an overdose of cobalt also causes the production of too many red cells and can interfere with thyroid gland function. However, there is a very wide margin of safety between what the body needs and the toxic levels that produce clinical problems and it's impossible to get an overdose of cobalt from normal eating and drinking.

COPPER

The presence of copper in plant and animal tissue was recognized over 150 years ago and it was shown to be essential for animals in 1928. Slowly, copper deficiency states were discovered and human copper deficiencies (associated with iron deficiency) were reported over 40 years ago and again in 1959. These reports were not confirmed and the subject of copper deficiency in humans was discounted only to be finally 'proved' in 1964.

Copper is a part of several enzymes and proteins but its exact role in the body is still ill-understood. More than 90 per cent of the copper in the blood is bound to a special protein called caeruloplasmin and it is certain that the body can't form red blood cells if it has no copper. Iron metabolism is closely linked to that of copper and a shortage of either element can cause a very similar-looking anaemia. In fact a person who is anaemic yet does not respond to the correct dose of iron could be short of copper. Copper is also needed for bone growth. Copper has a direct anti-bacterial and anti-viral effect and those who are deficient in it don't tan in the sun.

About 40 per cent of the copper we consume is absorbed and taken to the liver where it is stored and controlled. It is released from the liver during infection and stress. About 80 per cent of the copper we absorb is excreted in bile and only a tiny fraction (1 per cent) leaves the body in the urine.

Signs and symptoms of deficiency
There are nine well-recognized groups of people who may become short of copper.

1. Children who are severely malnourished or those who have prolonged diarrhoea.
2. Children who have severe malabsorption diseases.
3. Premature babies
4. Hospital patients being fed intravenously (if the 'feed' is too low in copper).
5. Children with a genetic defect of copper metabolism.
6. People who have been treated with special drugs to cure the toxicity of metals such as lead in their bodies.
7. People who live almost exclusively on highly processed foods which are very low in copper.
8. Some ill people who can't absorb copper normally.
9. People who have excessive amounts of zinc, cadmium, fluorine or molybdenum in their diets. These interfere with the absorption of copper and have been shown to produce deficiencies in humans and animals.

The earliest clinical signs of copper deficiency are: a lowering of the white blood cell count; a thinning of the bones (osteoporosis); and changes in hair texture and colour. Premature babies haven't had enough time in utero to build up their liver stores of copper, and babies weaned too early onto foods low in copper (cows' milk, for example, is rich in zinc which reduces the absorption of copper) start out in life at a disadvantage and fail to thrive, have diarrhoea, are pale, suffer from de-pigmentation of the hair and skin and have prominent, dilated superficial veins. Diarrhoea is a frequent result of copper deficiency in babies and in animals but it gets better quickly when they are given copper.

Menke's Steely Hair Syndrome is an inherited condition characterized by progressive degeneration of the nervous system in early infancy with the onset of convulsions at about three months and a fatal outcome later in infancy or childhood. The hair looks like the steel wool appearance of copper-deficient sheep. It is colourless, stubbly, stiff and like the steel wool used by decorators. A loss of hair colour and a loss of taste can be signs of copper deficiency in adults too. In one study about one third of the patients being treated with a drug called penicillamine had their failing sense of taste restored by taking copper supplements.

How to get enough

The richest dietary sources of copper are liver (especially of young animals), kidney, crustaceans and shellfish. Nuts, dried legumes, stone fruits, cocoa, yeast, beef extract and treacle are also fairly rich in copper. Unrefined cereal grains are a good source too. The copper content of leafy vegetables depends on the copper content of the soil on which they are grown and the poorest dietary sources are dairy products and refined sugar.

The water supply can make a significant impact on one's copper intake. Water flowing through copper pipes in soft water areas can be a meaningful source of dietary copper. It is thought that about 2–3mg of copper is required for health. More than 1mg can come from copper water pipes in soft water areas.

Although some of the medical profession and the public think it is ridiculous, some people who suffer from rheumatism wear copper bracelets and swear by their effectiveness. Copper may well be absorbed through sweaty skin—far more of many substances goes through the skin than was ever previously thought—and copper has now been shown to increase the anti-inflammatory powers of certain medicines and has slight anti-inflammatory properties itself. Copper-coated intra-uterine devices have been used for years and their increased effectiveness appears to relate to the tiny amounts of copper that dissolve off into the wall of the uterus.

Copper is available in food supplements and such preparations are used in certain cases of anaemia and even by some people who believe (though it isn't proven) that it will prevent their hair from greying.

FLUORINE
(active in the body as fluoride)

There is no doubt that fluoride is necessary for the healthy formation and growth of bones and teeth, yet because its addition to some domestic water supplies has been seen as an action of 'big brother' or the thin end of the wedge of unsolicited mass medication, it has received more than its fair share of bad publicity.

This is a pity because fluoride is known to be an essential trace element for animals and is likely to be essential for Man. Mice become anaemic and suffer from reduced fertility if they don't have enough fluoride; rats and chicks need it for normal growth and skeletal development; and humans need it for the growth of healthy teeth. Fluoride is especially necessary during childhood and more is retained by the body at this stage of life.

The debate about fluoride today centres around its use in preventing or reducing dental decay—which it does very effectively. It was in 1916 that a Colorado dentist first noticed that his patients had very few cavities in their teeth. The city's water supply was analysed and found to contain two parts per million of fluoride. It has since been found that the optimal level is one part per million so as to avoid the main effect of fluoride overdose (which some of this original dentist's patients had)—white mottling of the enamel of the teeth.

Today, many communities in the western world fluoridate their water supplies if the naturally-occurring level of fluoride is below one part per million. The results have been encouraging. Dental decay in such areas is lower by 50 per cent even in children who do nothing else to prevent decay. Those children who use a fluoride toothpaste and are very careful about their tooth cleaning often have no cavities at all. In fact a report from a British dental school recently stated that it was impossible to find enough dental decay in children in their area on which to teach their dental students about child tooth decay. They had to bus their students to non-fluoridated areas to find clinical material on which to teach.

Opponents of fluoridation are concerned about the principle of mass medication in everyone's domestic water whether they need the fluoride or not. They point to the dangers of overdose in the few people who drink lots of tea (a very rich source of fluoride); to the fact that some cows who have grazed on fluoride-rich pastures have become crippled; and to the ever-present danger of tooth mottling. Tooth decay, they argue, is a self-induced disease of western civilization, the answer to which is better tooth cleaning and fewer refined carbohydrate foods (sugar in particular)—not mass medication. There are also recent studies that suggest a link between fluoridation and certain birth defects, allergies and even cancers.

Signs and symptoms of deficiency
Children living in low-fluoride areas have more tooth decay than do those living in high-fluoride areas. Apart from this, no deficiency signs or symptoms are known in humans.

How to get enough
Most adults get enough fluoride, it is thought, simply by drinking tea, which is especially rich in the trace element. China tea is especially good in this respect. Six strong cups of tea contain about 3mg of fluoride. Every part per million of fluoride in our drinking water adds about 1mg of fluoride per day to our intake. If you want to know about your local drinking water ask your dentist or the local town hall.

Seafood is another good source of fluoride and many other foods contain some fluoride. Water alone, as we saw on page 17, can supply 10 per cent of one's fluoride needs, and water re-boiled time and again in a kettle can become dangerously rich in fluoride. Always empty the kettle at least once a day and refill it with fresh water.

Clearly people's fluoride intake can vary enormously. Someone who drinks no tea and lives in a non-fluoridated area will consume very little indeed, whereas heavy drinkers of strong tea living in a fluoridated area could consume about 10mg/day. The healthy intake is thought to be somewhere around the 5mg/day mark.

The only sign of overdose is mottling of the teeth. This takes the form of white flecks with or without brown patches or stripes. In very severe cases the teeth become pitted with tiny erosions. These changes are irreversible and are a serious cause of concern but only occur if fluoride is taken in excess.

IODINE

After iron, iodine was the second trace element known to be essential to Man, but even today, 150 years later, it is estimated that more than 200 million people throughout the world suffer from iodine deficiency diseases—mainly because they live in iodine-deficient soil areas. The main deficiency sign is a swelling of the thyroid gland in the neck (a goitre). Giving iodine to such people cures the goitre and adding iodized salt to their diet can prevent it occurring at all.

The only known functions of iodine are those connected with its presence in thyroid hormones. However, because these hormones are so vital to the body, iodine intake is essential. Thyroid hormones do several things:

- They control energy transformation through an effect on cellular oxygen consumption and heat production.
- They are essential for growth. Babies born with no thyroid tissue grow up dwarfed and have delayed development if untreated.
- They are necessary for reproductive function. Children born with no thyroid gland and who are not treated with thyroid hormones are sterile, and young animals from whom the thyroid gland has been removed remain infantile.
- They are vital for the functioning of the nerves and muscles.
- They are necessary for normal hair and skin growth.
- They are needed for cellular metabolic processes of many kinds. It has been estimated that more than 100 enzymes are affected by the giving of thyroid hormones and protein synthesis (the build up of tissue for growth and repair) also depends on these hormones.

So clearly any defect in the production of thyroid hormones can play havoc with the body's normal functioning and in turn the body's ability to produce these hormones depends on there being an adequate supply of iodine in the diet.

Signs and symptoms of deficiency
The main one is an enlarged thyroid gland in the neck (a goitre). The degree of enlargement can vary greatly from a small, hardly perceivable, swelling to a gigantic one which obstructs the breathing passages. The person becomes slowed mentally and physically and feels low or even frankly depressed. The skin is dry and the features coarse. The thyroid gland enlarges as it tries desperately to extract what iodine there is in the body and over-works to try to produce enough thyroid hormones. If you ever have any of these symptoms, see a doctor.

But it's not only a lack of iodine that can cause such an underactive thyroid gland—substances known as goitrogens can do so too. These are naturally-occurring chemicals which prevent the thyroid gland from using what iodine there is in the body. It's likely that there are many more goitrogens than we currently realize but plants of the brassica family (for example swedes and cabbages) and excessive intakes of cobalt or manganese are known to interfere with iodine usage in the body in some circumstances.

Women appear to be more susceptible than men to a shortage of iodine, especially during pregnancy and breast-feeding. Signs of thyroid hormone problems are most likely at puberty and during adolescence.

How to get enough
The best source of iodine is seafood and a meal or two containing fish or another seafood every week should keep most people healthy in this respect. Seaweed, kelp and laverbread are other rich sources of iodine. The next most valuable sources of iodine are iodized table salt, sea salt and fish liver oils. It is known that boiling fish removes much of its valuable iodine so other methods of preparation are preferable. The effects on iodine of the freezing and thawing of fish have not yet been finally worked out.

Commercial preparations of seaweed, kelp and carageen (Irish moss) are available in health food shops if one wants to supplement one's dietary intake of iodine.

IRON

This is hardly a 'trace' element in the true sense of the word because it is relatively plentiful in the body (it is the most abundant of the trace elements) and is not present in 'trace' amounts. It's worth considering here though because its metabolism is so intimately tied up with that of other trace elements and because it has been studied so extensively and therefore provides insights into the workings of the other trace elements.

Although iron has been known to be essential and of therapeutic value since ancient times, there's still a lot we don't know about it and there's still considerable controversy about how much we need, the definition of iron deficiency and its effects and the best way of treating it. But having said this we still know a lot about iron and more money is spent on remedying this element's deficiency than on any other.

Iron's main function in the body is its vital role in the structure of the red blood cells, without which the rest of the body's cells wouldn't get an oxygen supply. About two thirds of the body's 4 grams of iron are tied up in haemoglobin, the red blood cell pigment. Some is stored in the liver and yet more in the muscles as myoglobin. The bone marrow has a supply too because it is here that the red blood cells are made and as each cell lives for only 120 days there is a constant demand for new iron to make new haemoglobin. Some of the body's iron is re-used from the broken down red cells but some needs to be taken in the diet.

But for all our knowledge iron deficiency is still an extremely common condition throughout even the westernized world where, one would imagine, everyone had access to healthy foods. In fact it is generally agreed that iron deficiency is the most widespread nutritional deficiency world-wide. In Third World countries much of the iron that people eat is biologically unavailable because it is bound in the intestine by phytic acid (a substance found in fibre-rich cereal foods). Also, millions of people suffer from intestinal worms and parasites that render them anaemic and incapable of producing enough red blood cells to keep up with the loss. In the western world people are still ignorant of which foods are rich in iron and they also don't absorb much of what they do eat. Only about 10 per cent of the iron we consume is available to the body and some foods yield less than 5 per cent of their iron in the intestine. Meat and fish are better sources than plants but the ability to absorb iron varies from person to person and within any one person according to his iron status at the time. A normal child who is iron-deficient can have double the normal adult absorption of iron from his intestine.

Iron absorption has been extensively studied yet is still ill-understood. Iron in food occurs in a number of forms and inorganic iron is complexed by starch, fibre, protein and phosphate-rich substances such as phytic acid and vitallin. Because of the affinity of phytates for iron, foods rich in phytates decrease iron absorption. Iron absorption is enhanced by including meat in the diet. Orange juice taken with a meal enhances iron absorption and excessive supplementation with zinc and copper inhibits it. Tea and coffee are also now known to reduce the absorption of this vital mineral.

In addition to these problem areas, many of us in the West are losing blood on a long term basis and its natural replacement reduces our body stores of iron which, if not replaced in turn, can make us ill. Women in their childbearing years are at greatest risk from iron deficiency because unless they are eating an iron-rich diet they simply can't make up the iron lost in the menstrual blood loss each month. This problem is made worse if they have had several pregnancies, especially in quick succession, because the foetus needs considerable amounts of iron (if it is to grow normally in the uterus). Breast-feeding too makes further demands on a woman's iron stores. To combat these problems women seem to have been designed by nature to absorb iron more effectively from their food than have men.

But it's not only women who are susceptible to iron deficiency. Millions of people of both sexes in the western world have piles (haemorrhoids) that bleed from time to time; some have a duodenal or gastric ulcer that may bleed a little every day; others take aspirin or other anti-arthritic drugs regularly which cause a blood loss from the stomach; and of course anyone who has had an operation or an accident at which blood was lost will have to make up the deficit and this will require iron.

Vitamin C is known to improve iron absorption and because many people are short of this vitamin this could be another reason why they are iron-deficient. Copper (almost entirely removed from many foods in refining) is an important co-factor in iron metabolism and is essential if iron is to make healthy blood. As we saw on page 45 it's easy to get too little of this vital element.

Of course anyone eating a poor diet, such as the elderly, the very poor or malnourished and fanatical slimmers, can simply be getting so little iron in any form that it is easy for them to go short. Vegetarians too can become iron-deficient because although they eat a lot of iron-containing foods they don't eat meat and fish which are the best sources and encourage the absorption of iron from other foods. There are lots of vegetarian sources of iron though, the best being soya beans, yeast extract and almonds and most vegetarians, aware that they need to be especially vigilant over their diet, eat a lot of foods containing vitamin C which help the absorption of whatever iron there is.

Signs and symptoms of deficiency

Millions of people throughout the world are mildly iron-deficient yet don't realize it. They are simply more tired than they should be, have more infections than they should have and generally lack energy. Anaemia is often a main finding and iron deficiency anaemia is the commonest type of anaemia in the western world. As the anaemia becomes more severe the person becomes physically and mentally tired by the slightest exertion, and even eventually breathless at rest. Having said this, it is perfectly possible to be iron-deficient without being anaemic.

Angina pectoris can occur as the heart finds it difficult to extract enough oxygen from the blood it receives and some iron-deficient people complain of a 'poor circulation', especially in their legs. Evidence is accumulating that suggests that voluntary activity is reduced in experimental animals with mild iron deficiency in which severe anaemia has not yet developed. Although this is still controversial, the finding has been supported by one human study. If this is confirmed it could totally question our current views on optimal iron levels. This would be of special interest to haematologists who assume that unless iron deficiency produces anaemia there is little or no effect on a person's health. It's also interesting that mild iron deficiency (producing only a mild anaemia) increases the absorption of the potentially toxic elements lead and cadmium.

Iron deficiency in childhood impairs learning ability and concentration and produces sleep disturbances and behaviour problems.

How to get enough

Although the best sources of iron are meat, eggs and fish, in the UK other foods supply the majority of people's iron. Bread, cereals, potatoes and vegetables supply two thirds of our iron, and meat and fish the remaining third. This is probably because meat and fish are relatively expensive and because we eat more bread and vegetables. Animal sources of iron don't have to be expensive though—black pudding, sprats, liver and sardines are all very rich sources that are also fairly cheap. Green, leafy vegetables and whole grains are also good sources of iron but, contrary to popular belief, spinach is not a particularly rich source.

The recommended daily requirements for iron are 10mg for men, 12mg for women and 18mg for children and women in their reproductive years.

As well as taking iron in our food it is also widely available in the form of commercial preparations. Iron tablets are the most popular but can cause tummy upsets if not taken with food. They can also cause constipation, especially in the elderly. Iron-fortified tonics and tonic wines are a good source of iron, and molasses and powdered liver are both excellent easy-to-take sources. Because iron is so poorly absorbed, efforts have been made with certain iron tablets to mimic the body's iron absorption mechanism. These are the so-called chelated iron tablets in which the iron is coated with protein to aid absorption and reduce its irritant effects. As was pointed out earlier, excessive usage of iron-rich supplements restricts the absorption of zinc. Because of this, and because it is now known that some people aren't able naturally to restrict the absorption of excessive iron (as most of us are) it makes sense to avoid long term iron supplements without medical advice.

Undoubtedly the best way to prevent iron deficiency is to eat a diet rich in iron-containing foods and to see your doctor if you think you have any cause for iron loss, such as heavy periods, perhaps from using an IUD; unexplained upper abdominal pains which could be due to an ulcer; obvious blood loss from anywhere; the long term use of aspirin or anti-arthritic drugs; bleeding haemorrhoids; after an operation or accident at which you lost blood; or if you have been repeatedly pregnant or have breast-fed for long periods. There's very little point in eating a better diet if you continue to lose available blood (with its iron) and do nothing about it.

MANGANESE

This is a rather enigmatic but nevertheless essential trace element which is present in the soft tissues, pituitary gland, liver and kidney (in decreasing order of concentration in the body). It appears to be necessary for intra-uterine growth, growth generally, the normal functioning of nervous tissue, and for many of the body's 'activator' systems. It may be important for a mother's instinctual feelings for her child (by its action on certain 'maternal' hormones), for the formation of thyroid hormones, and for the production of nucleic acids (special proteins that make up the genetic code in each cell). A healthy adult's body contains between 12–20mg of manganese, about a fifth of the amount of copper.

Studies have suggested that manganese could be useful in treating schizophrenia, and one study found that diabetics had low blood manganese levels compared with non-diabetics. In the case of the schizophrenics it is claimed that those who have a high level of copper in their blood are improved by taking a combination of zinc and manganese.

The body of the average adult appears to lose 4mg a day of this element, so presumably to keep in balance we need to absorb the same amount.

Signs and symptoms of deficiency
Apart from the link with diabetes mentioned above, no deficiency states

have been described in humans, though animal deficiencies are well-documented. It has been suggested that older men may be manganese-deficient and that atherosclerosis could partly be caused by manganese deficiency. The enzymes that manganese activates are known to be essential for the utilization of vitamin C and certain B vitamins, and myasthenia gravis has been found to respond to manganese given with a high protein diet, vitamin E and all the B-vitamins.

How to get enough
Leafy vegetables, nuts, spices and whole grains are the main dietary sources of manganese, and tea is an especially good source. One cupful of tea contains 1mg of the element. Because most people in the UK eat so much refined food from which most of the manganese has been removed it's just as well that they drink a lot of tea to make up for this dietary loss.

MOLYBDENUM

Molybdenum has for some time been known to be essential for plants which need to fix atmospheric nitrogen and use it for their own metabolism but its role in animal nutrition is still something of a mystery. It is thought to be essential for all mammals because it is found in almost all their tissues and certain beneficial actions are well proven.

Like fluorine, molybdenum appears to prevent dental caries and it has been speculatively linked to oesophageal cancer in certain parts of the world. For example, parts of South Africa and China where this cancer is rife have very molybdenum-deficient vegetation. US studies of molybdenum-deficient areas have found the same link. Sexual impotence in older men too has been linked to molybdenum deficiency. Iron metabolism requires the action of an enzyme called xanthine oxidase which in turn is known to be molybdenum-dependent. This same enzyme is also needed for the body to break down certain proteins to uric acid. Only one study has made such a link but it is a convincing one—abnormally high levels of blood uric acid (producing gout and uric acid stones in the urine) were linked with a high level of molybdenum in the local soil of a particular community in Armenia.

Molybdenum is an essential element in the enzyme system that inactivates sulphites, bisulphites and metabisulphites. Allergy to these components of our diet may be in part due to a molybdenum deficiency.

Signs and symptoms of deficiency

One recent report describes the accidental development of molybdenum deficiency in a hospitalized patient maintained on an intravenous 'feed' ultimately found to be low in molybdenum. Symptoms were easily reversed once the problem was detected. These included heart beat irregularities, irritability, coma, and a marked alteration in the metabolism of uric acid.

How to get enough

Although the element is difficult to measure it is thought that a wide variety of foods contain it. There is no consensus as to what the 'ideal' intake is. Whole grains, wheat germ, sunflower seeds, liver, lima beans, canned beans and soya beans are all good sources.

SELENIUM

This is one of the classic examples of a trace element which was for years thought to be only toxic and which today is known to be essential for life within a very small range of intake. The amount of selenium a food contains (and thus how much an animal or a person gets) depends almost entirely on the amount of selenium in the soil on which it was grown. It is now widely recognized that the earth's crust has many low-selenium areas which in turn produce low-selenium water supplies. Low soil levels produce a condition called nutritional muscular dystrophy or 'white muscle disease' in animals but selenium has many other effects too. It is essential for normal liver function and is intimately involved in maintaining the activity of white blood cells as scavengers of foreign micro-organisms. It also protects against the toxic effects of cadmium and laboratory tests on animals show that it protects against high mercury in tuna fish. In all species it works closely with vitamin E. There are suggestions, as yet not adequately confirmed, that it reduces the chances of contracting all types of cancer. Several studies have found that communities where selenium intake is low have higher than expected cancer rates.

Males seem to need more selenium than do females and breast milk contains up to six times as much selenium as cows' milk and twice as much vitamin E. Australian researchers have linked selenium deficiency to the tragic condition known as 'cot death' in which an otherwise normal baby dies in its sleep for some mysterious reason. Extensive studies in China have shown that a deficiency in selenium is one important factor in the high incidence of heart failure in young children in some areas.

Although there are suspicions that a recurrent viral infection is also involved the protective effect of minute oral supplements of selenium has been proven.

A disadvantage of selenium appears to be its ability to increase dental caries in children under the age of 12. Heavy consumption of selenium appears to reduce the protective effect of fluoride.

Animal studies have found that selenium reduces high blood pressure and when combined with vitamin E it reduces angina pectoris.

Selenium-deficient animals don't reproduce and selenium has been found to be one ingredient of male semen—in fact half of a man's body stores of selenium are found in the testes and seminal glands. Selenium is also part of the enzyme system that controls the production of the naturally-occurring hormone-like substances called prostaglandins. Since these have extremely widespread functions throughout the body selenium may turn out to be even more important than it at first appears.

Signs and symptoms of deficiency
See the above section about the heart effects. Also, there are tentative claims that a selenium deficiency produced by low selenium intravenous 'feeds' produces muscular pain.

How to get enough
This isn't known as yet because the same foods grown on different soils of the world vary greatly in how much selenium they contain. However, brewer's yeast, garlic, eggs, fish and liver are good sources. Animal foods are generally richer than vegetable foods. Unfortunately, selenium is easily lost in processing—for example, brown rice has 15 times the selenium content of white rice and wholemeal bread contains twice that of white bread.

There is increasing evidence that people living in some areas don't get enough selenium partly because so many areas of the world (including the UK) are low-selenium soil regions.

ZINC

There is probably more known about zinc than about any of the other trace elements except perhaps iron and iodine. It is the second most plentiful trace element after iron. Like copper, the biological role of this element was established well over a century ago but as with so many of the long-known trace elements it wasn't until the '60s that the medical and scientific communities began to realize how important it was to Man.

Zinc is important because it is essential for the production and efficient working of more than 40 zinc-containing enzymes. It is also crucial in the synthesis of the DNA and RNA at the heart of every living cell. There are now literally thousands of learned papers in the medical and scientific literature on the various actions of zinc, and it is totally accepted along with iron and iodine in the US as being essential in many clinical situations.

Research has found that zinc is crucial for growth prenatally (during pregnancy) and afterwards. Maternal zinc deficiency in rats produces a wide range of minor and major congenital malformations involving especially the nervous system and the skeleton. Only a brief period of zinc deficiency is needed to produce these effects. Zinc deficiency around the time of birth retards growth and subsequent learning ability.

A fully grown adult's body contains about 2g of zinc (about half the body's iron content and 20 times its copper content) and almost all of this comes from food. Only about 20–30 per cent of the zinc we consume is absorbed, and zinc from animal protein is much better absorbed than that from vegetables. Rather as with iron, the amount absorbed from food depends on the person's zinc status at the time. Zinc given orally can be detected in the blood 15 minutes later, the blood level reaching a peak in four hours.

Signs and symptoms of deficiency
A person can become short of zinc for several reasons. A dietary insufficiency of zinc is probably the commonest cause; a person may eat foods low in animal protein, and much zinc is lost in food processing. Fans of processed foods may be unable to get enough zinc however much food they eat. Having said this, there's little evidence that most people are zinc-deficient as judged by many nutritional experts' notions of adequate amounts. However, as with so many of the trace elements, there is a very substantial debate as to what really does constitute a safe intake.

It is now known that certain components of the diet inhibit the absorption of zinc—the most important being the phytic acid found in whole-grain cereals and some vegetable proteins such as soya beans.

While such components are known to be important in farm animals, their exact significance in Man is not yet clear. This is because their effects as zinc antagonists depend on the calcium content of their diet. Whilst a lot more research needs to be done on all this it makes sense to suppose that the absorption of zinc from a diet simultaneously rich in calcium and phytic acid may be reduced. Certain diseases and illnesses alter the absorption of zinc from the intestine. Any condition that causes the intestinal contents to rush through can mean that too little is absorbed and in a condition called acrodermatitis enteropathica (see over) there is an inherited inability to absorb zinc. More rarely, conditions can arise in which a person loses too much zinc and an abnormal loss of zinc in the urine is now increasingly reported in many illnesses.

Probably the second most common cause for zinc deficiency after too low an intake is the increased need for more at periods of greater demand. We know that during periods of rapid growth (childhood and adolescence), during pregnancy, whilst breast-feeding and when the body is healing burns and wounds, the need for zinc rises substantially and it is easy to go short, even with a 'good' diet.

Diabetics have low body zinc levels and zinc is certainly needed for the storage and release of insulin. The elderly are at risk of zinc deficiency because they seem to absorb it less well, and heavy drinkers also absorb the element badly. Several drugs, including oral contraceptives, reduce zinc levels and soft water flowing through copper pipes dissolves off copper which antagonizes zinc absorption in the body.

The signs and symptoms of deficiency are many and depend on the age of the individual, how quickly the deficiency comes on, how long it has been there, and on the circumstances in which the deficiency occurs. Table 6 shows the commonest features of zinc deficiency.

Studies have found, for example, that maternal zinc deficiency may be a factor in the production of babies with anencephaly in areas where this distressing abnormality of the skull is commoner than expected. Adult women suffering from acrodermatitis enteropathica also tend to have babies with a high incidence of congenital malformations. Many experts are increasingly concerned that baby foods and infant diets generally don't produce nearly enough zinc for the optimal intake of a baby and studies have found that growth is delayed in such children. Nutritional dwarfism has been studied in Egypt and iron and zinc have been shown to play a crucial role.

Once growth is complete the nutritional requirements for zinc are much lower and the effects of zinc deficiency are less severe except during pregnancy and while breast-feeding. However, zinc probably speeds wound

Table 6. Zinc deficiency signs and symptoms

Loss of appetite	Diarrhoea
Slowing of growth	Poor or reduced sex drive
Eating of dirt or strange substances by children (pica)	Poor wound healing
Loss of taste	Mental depression Increased susceptibility to infenctions
Loss of smell	(Possibly white flecks in the nails)
Delayed sexual maturity in children	
Loss of hair	

Development of skin rashes with scaly lesions around the mouth, eyes, vagina, nose and on areas that suffer even the mildest abrasion.

healing in surgical patients and leg ulcers heal quicker too if zinc supplements are taken. Unfortunately, the dietary status of many in-patients in hospital is made worse by the poor zinc levels of institutional food: by the withholding of food prior to operations; by the surgery itself which causes more zinc than normal to be lost in the urine; and as a result of the increased needs for zinc at the site of the wound for the healing process. For all of these reasons a zinc-balanced individual could become zinc-deficient after an operation unless he took more zinc-containing foods or zinc as a supplement.

It is now realized that the body puts out a lot of zinc in the urine with infectious hepatitis, with burns, after multiple injuries (for example, a car crash), after fractures of major bones, in out-of-control diabetes and during starvation. People on water tablets (diuretics) also lose a lot of zinc in their urine.

A rare but interesting type of zinc deficiency is known as acrodermatitis enteropathica. This is an inherited condition in which there is a loss of hair, skin lesions and diarrhoea. Symptoms start in infancy, though if the infant is breast-fed they are usually delayed until after weaning. In the classical untreated condition the course is downhill and the child dies in early childhood. However, treatment with zinc produces a dramatic improvement and the child lives. Such children may have to be given zinc supplements permanently because of their inability to absorb the zinc they do eat. Both children suffering from the untreated form of this condition and zinc-deficient animals have been found to have a much higher than expected incidence of infections generally and zinc is now definitely accepted as being essential for the combatting of infections.

How to get enough
With modern food processing removing zinc from even zinc-plentiful foods there's a danger that many of the population and especially those at risk (outlined above)—are zinc-deficient at any one time. Many US experts agree that zinc deficiency is enormously widespread even among the so-called 'healthy' population. An adult man needs about 15–20mg/day but the pregnant and breast-feeding woman needs more (probably double this amount).

The best sources of dietary zinc are seafoods, but meat generally is a good source too. Whole grains, nuts, peas and beans are rich in zinc but not in forms that are as readily absorbed as from meat, dairy produce and green vegetables. Zinc tablets are available to supplement a possibly zinc-deficient diet. People's tolerance to zinc supplements varies in different circumstances, even within the same person. For example, tolerance to dietary zinc is not high in late pregnancy and there are even suggestions from India that zinc supplements taken at this time can increase perinatal mortality or even cause the foetus to die. As far as is known, zinc is well tolerated at other times.

There's little doubt that many of us living in the West, and eating what we think of as healthy foods, are short of zinc, especially during rapid growth periods and in the circumstances outlined above.

One exciting but not life-saving application for zinc has been in acne. Zinc taken orally seems to reduce the number of eruptions.

Because zinc is essential for human reproduction and sexual maturation and is probably necessary for optimal fertility in men it was (irresponsibly) claimed to be good for one's sex life. Certainly some impotent young men have been cured by taking zinc daily for 4–5 months but as to zinc being a kind of aphrodisiac, the evidence is simply not there. One study found that zinc produced beneficial effects in men suffering from an inflammation of the prostate gland. This can be a very long term and nagging infection which is annoying for the sufferer so any simple dietary aid is very welcome.

TRACE ELEMENT OVERDOSE

The vast majority of people eating healthily are very unlikely to consume too much of any one trace element but it can happen in one of several ways. First, the person may eat a cranky, unbalanced diet consisting of a few foods very rich in a particular element or two. Second, because of human errors in food processing a food can be contaminated with too much of a trace element. Third, an individual could take too much of a trace element supplement by ignoring the manufacturer's instructions. This latter is foolish because, as we have seen already, many of the trace elements compete with each other in the intestine. Taking a lot of one (on the basis that it'll do more good or do it quicker) could seriously alter the balance of several others.

Normal eating, as far as we know, never produces an overdose of the useful trace elements but increasing research is suggesting that even normal diets in certain parts of the world can contain toxic levels of particular toxic elements which can alter the metabolism of the useful ones. The commonest toxic trace elements that act in this way are cadmium, lead and mercury.

Although it obviously makes sense to eat food that is as 'natural' and unrefined as possible, the most important thing is to eat a balance of many different foods. Food faddists eating a poor selection even of natural, unrefined foods can all too easily become deficient in one or more trace element.

INDEX